Acupuncture Treatment for Glaucoma:

Clinically Proven Methods to Recover & Preserve Optic Nerve Health

DR. ANDY ROSENFARB, ND, L.Ac.

MEDICAL DISCLAIMER:
The following information is intended for general information purposes only.
Individuals should always see their health care provider before administering any
suggestions made in this book. Any application of the material set forth in the
following pages is at the reader's discretion and is his or her sole responsibility.

Contents

Introduction

Andy Rosenfarb specializes in treating degenerative eye conditions with Acupuncture, Chinese Medicine, and Naturopathic Medicine. Dr. Rosenfarb has been practicing since 1996 and has worked with thousands of patients from around the world with various degenerative eye conditions. He has become the leading authority in the field of Ophthalmic Acupuncture and Naturopathic Ophthalmology.

In addition to Glaucoma, other common eye conditions treated by Dr. Rosenfarb include Macular Degeneration, Retinitis Pigmentosa, Usher's Syndrome, Diabetic Retinopathies and optic nerve Atrophy.

Our Clinical objective for treating each patient is this:

1) Improve and recover lost vision, if possible.

2) Preserve vision long-term and help you keep what you've got.

My goal in this book is to give you a little information about the kind of work I do for those dealing with glaucoma – or those who have loved ones diagnosed with glaucoma. I'll make some general suggestions for supplements, lifestyle, and nutrition which may help slow the progression of your condition, by preserving the health and function of the optic nerve. If you have any questions beyond what is covered here, please feel free to contact our office at your convenience to further discuss your situation and what options might be available to you.

Glaucoma

Glaucoma is a "silent" disease that can go asymptomatic for many years and slowly steal your vision. With most cases, there is no pain signal to alert you that something is wrong. By the time you figure out that something is happening, the disease process may have already progressed to a moderate or advanced state.

At that point, you are typically told by your eye doctor that you have glaucoma with elevated eye pressure and or normal tension glaucoma. Your doctor will most likely prescribe medications (eye drops) or surgical procedures (like SLT or trabeculectomy) in an attempt to control your eye pressure. Once the eye pressure(s) are down and within a safe range, it becomes a "wait and see" game. The million-dollar question that we need to now consider is this, "Why do people still keep losing their vision when the pressure is kept in a relatively normal range?"

If glaucoma was only an eye pressure issue, then once the pressure is controlled, theoretically that should arrest progressive vision loss. In reality, we know that is often not the case and people continue to lose vision even though the pressure is controlled with surgery and medication.

From my perspective, there are three main factors that typically drive the degenerative vision loss process. These factors are not well understood and are typically overlooked and/or ignored by conventional medicine. These factors include:

1- Oxidative Stress

2- Inflammation

3- Poor Circulation

Oxidative Stress comes from free radical damage. Free Radicals are highly reactive atoms with unpaired electrons that (if they get out of control) will go around destroying healthy cells and tissues.

Excessive Free Radicals accelerate aging and neurodegeneration. Most health care providers agree that for most eye conditions (and other neurodegenerative conditions), "antioxidant" vitamins and herbs may be helpful.

We have found that the absolute best type of antioxidants for eye protection are called Carotenoid antioxidants. We can even test your specific Carotenoid antioxidant levels. We do this for all our eye patients and it lets us know if each patient has sufficient levels of protective Carotenoid antioxidants in their bodies.

Other common antioxidants include Vitamin A, C, and E, Zinc, Selenium, Lutein, and Zeaxanthin and Meso-Zeaxanthin as well as fruits, vegetables, leafy greens, etc. These are all packed with beneficial antioxidants and should be consumed as well for additional protection against free radical damage. Consuming these foods with high antioxidant properties helps to reduce oxidative stress and protects the body from accelerated degeneration and vision loss.

We also want to stay hydrated and eat clean, organic foods. Water is a powerful antioxidant and dehydration can exacerbate the damaging effects of inflammation and oxidative stress. I suggest drinking a large glass of water first thing in the morning and then again throughout the day - between meals.

There are other known factors that can accelerate oxidative stress. These are usually things that we know are inherently "bad" for our health including smoking, alcohol, refined sugar, junk food, and most drugs and medications. Consuming these products simply puts more garbage in your body that will rob us of healthy vitality, as well as deteriorate our overall health. It will also accelerate neurodegenerative conditions like Glaucoma.

Acute intense stress episodes and prolonged emotional stress can also accelerate oxidative stress and negatively impact our health and vision. If an individual tends to be quite anxious, worries a lot, angers easily, gets depressed often, etc., this can eventually have a severe negative impact on vision. Learning to manage stress is critical to slow the process of these kinds of diseases. Some of us are just wired as Type-A, high stressed individuals and others just seem to have an easier time letting things roll off our shoulders. Managing stress is one of the best things we can do to help control the rate of progressive loss. We need to constantly evaluate our stress levels and work to improve our ability to handle stress. Making these kinds of positive lifestyle changes will help reduce the oxidative stress load in the body.

There are ways to subjectively and objectively check oxidative stress in your body. One way is just by simply looking at people. We know we all age as time goes on, but there is the one thing that we can see that gives us an indicator of our level of oxidative stress - our skin! That's right ... our skin. Sometimes you might notice someone that looks a little bit more wrinkly than usual - they most definitely have elevated oxidative stress. Usually, these folks are highly stressed, smokers, alcohol drinkers, on a lot of medications and/or those who have spent too much time in the sun. Stress and poor diet can cause this kind of oxidative skin damage as well. If a person has a lot of premature age-spots, that is another indicator of oxidative stress that is damaging the skin and most likely other areas of the body as well.

I always work with my patients to try to identify the presence and degree of oxidative stress, and we then work to reduce oxidative stress with good supplements, fruits and vegetables – and by reducing the lifestyle habits that may accelerate oxidative stress. The first signs we often see is improved skin health.

Oxidative stress not only attacks our skin, it is also breaks down the optic nerve, retina, lens (cataracts), heart and the brain. Oxidative stress is a systemic factor that accelerates degeneration and robs our health We need to take a holistic approach to measure and manage excessive systemic oxidation levels to slow (or arrest) the progression of vision loss. Ultra-Violet (UV) rays come from the sun and is a form of radiation that causes oxidative stress on the eyes.

Blue light is another form of light that can cause stress to our eyes and comes from the sun and from computer screens (and smartphones). We need to always wear protective eyewear to reduce exposure and potential oxidative damage from UV and Blue light radiation.

Other factors that can cause oxidative stress include smoking, drugs/meds, alcohol, obesity, and stress. Fried foods and processed "junk" foods are the most highly oxidative and damaging to the eye, brain and optic nerve.

Inflammation is a significant driving factor that both causes and accelerates vision loss. Acute and chronic inflammation can come from a host of factors including trauma, excessive stress, poor diet, pollution, heavy metals, pesticides, GMO's, chronic allergies, infections, autoimmune processes, medications, UV-Light, etc. Many of my patients ask me about taking anti-inflammatory vitamins, herbs, and supplements for their eye condition. Although they may be helpful in some cases, it's a better practice to identify the source of the inflammation. After we identify the causative factor(s), we can then work to control the inflammatory processes and help keep that heat from damaging healthy tissue. Inflammation is another factor that often is ignored or overlooked – but critical to long-term vision preservation. In a comprehensive treatment plan, it's very important to assess and correct underlying inflammatory markers. We need to figure out specifically where the inflammation is coming from and control it so that it won't accelerate optic nerve degeneration which can lead to vision loss.

We have developed acupuncture methods that are highly effective in helping to control chronic inflammation that can increase optic nerve damage and accelerate vision loss.

Poor Circulation: Many neurodegenerative conditions (including glaucoma) can be affected by reduced blood flow. How do we know if there is systemic poor blood flow? If you notice that your hands and feet get cold often, that may be an indication that the peripheral blood flow is not good. You may not be very active. You start to get cracked, split nails or maybe a toenail fungus. This tells us that the circulation to our hands and feet is not as good as it used to be, or as good as it could be.

Exercise, certain herbs and supplements (like fish oil, ginkgo, ginger, and turmeric) and acupuncture can help improve peripheral blood flow and maintain healthy retinal and optic nerve function. Again, we need to figure out what the cause is for the impaired blood flow and address that. Herbs and supplements can help, but we need to get to the root cause of the impaired blood flow. Some of these factors may include anemia (low blood volume), low blood pressure, adrenal fatigue, low electrolytes, medications, cardiovascular disease, low body fat, general vascular deregulation, and stress.

Why do we need to optimize blood flow to the retina and optic nerve? All cells of our body need a constant supply of oxygen, nutrients and they need to eliminate waste material. All cells are mini-versions of us and like we need to breathe in air/oxygen, eat and eliminate waste, the cells in our body depend on adequate circulation in order to function and stay healthy. Cells need to breathe and eat food in order to grow, repair and produce energy. The eyes need micro and macronutrients (proteins, fats, sugars, and carbs) and vitamins and minerals to repair and stay healthy.

We use unique acupuncture methods as one of the best ways to maintain proper blood flow to the eyes. These methods have been scientifically proven and confirmed to increase blood flow to the eyes.

The primary goal of our acupuncture therapy is to improve the blood flowing to the optic nerve and retina. Again, conventional medicine focuses exclusively on lowering eye pressure (IOP) and has no current treatment that targets long-term preservation, health, and function of the optic nerve itself. There's no drug or surgery to help improve the blood flow to the optic nerve, control inflammation, and oxidative stress. Acupuncture is one of the safest and most effective methods to increase and maintain blood flow to the optic nerve and preserve vision.

Glaucoma patients who choose integrative care (conventional and acupuncture) seem to do the best with maintaining their vision. We've had patients under care for over 20 years who have successfully preserved their vision or at least dramatically slowed the progress.

The combination of using conventional approach to manage eye pressure coupled with the acupuncture and targeted nutrition appears to provide the best possible long-term outcome for patients.

Systematic Nature of Glaucoma

Glaucoma can be caused by many underlying conditions, most common being Autonomic Nervous System (ANS) dysfunction and autoimmune (AI) disease. At least half the cases present with normal-tension glaucoma (NTG) seems to be rooted in systemic auto-immune dysfunction. This is something that I have observed over the last 20 years in working with NTG patients.

Clinically, with these cases where there seems to be autoimmune, we need to control the overactive immune system from damaging the retina and optic nerve.

I suspect that with many of these NTG cases, the immune system may be attacking the optic nerve - causing progressive vision loss.

There are so many cases where the IOP medications simply are not enough to prevent vision loss. Patients are put on meds and vision loss continues even if the eye pressure is within normal range.

Remember, eye pressure is just one of many factors that cause optic nerve degeneration. Even with normal eye pressure, we STILL can lose vision.

The conventional glaucoma medical community has not yet reached the point where they have fully embraced this way of thinking in terms of considering these "other factors" that drive progressive optic nerve damage. Integrative Medical practices treat BOTH the cause (autonomic nervous system dysfunction, auto-immune, etc.) and the effects of vision loss (the eyes) and offers the best possible outcome for patients.

So, what is Auto-Immune (AI)?

AI is when the body's immune system attacks its own tissue like it would any foreign invaders like viruses, bacteria, fungus, yeast, cancer cells, etc. I suspect that in some cases the body creates antibodies that attack the optic nerve and retinal cells which are similar to how the body creates antibodies that attack the thyroid (Hashimoto's). Another example is when the body attacks the joints, as in rheumatoid arthritis. We know that antibodies can develop and attack the nerves and brain causing conditions like Multiple Sclerosis (MS). We need to start considering these factors and other possible underlying causes.

Conventional Medicine for

Treating Eye Disease

Conventional medicine tends to look at eye diseases like glaucoma as isolated organ (eye) pathologies – just a disease of the eyes. The condition is said to be a "natural aging process" that can either stabilize or get worse.

Conventional medical approaches to treating eye diseases include using corrective glasses/contacts for refractive issues, oral medications (steroids and antibiotics), eye drops, surgical procedures. Current medical research is focusing on stem cell and gene therapy.

Chinese medicine considers the whole body and the eye condition as it relates to the entire living organism. Again, we are looking both locally (eyes) and systemically (underlying cause). When my patients come to see me for eye conditions, I explain that we need to start a systemic evaluation to figure out the underlying causes for their condition. This is not like auto-mechanics, where we swap out interchangeable car parts. We are dealing with a living organism that works more like an ecosystem or a garden, rather than a machine.

Vision can be affected by all systems of the body - immune, circulatory, respiratory, etc. In Chinese medicine, a lot of eye conditions are related to liver and kidney dysfunction. That does not mean someone is having liver or kidney failure, rather the more functional aspect of these organs. The liver manages much of the detoxification process, stores glucose (as glucagon fuel) and helps manage oxidative stress. The kidneys deal with the fluids, electrolytes, and in Chinese Medicine, deal with the central nervous system (spine brain, eyes). So, we need to support these systems in terms of function.

The approach Chinese Medicine takes is relatively holistic. We look at your eyes as well as try to figure out what is causing your condition. "Genetics" and "Old Age" are not caused. It's a circumstance or a predisposition. It simply means that your healthcare provider may not have an understanding regarding the underlying cause for your condition.

There is more to medicine than drugs and surgery. We can use therapies like acupuncture, supplements, lifestyle modifications, improving nutrition and diet, stress management, exercise, and meditation. For many of these conditions, there is simply no conventional treatment. As we have discussed, conventional medical treatment for glaucoma focuses solely on controlling eye pressure. Controlling IOP does not guarantee sustained optic nerve health. We need to dig deeper and find the true root cause(s) of the various forms of glaucoma.

Stress and Vision

Stress management is a major part of our program and critical to long-term vision preservation. Simply stated, stress will rob your vision!

The majority of eye patients I've worked with say that stressful situations usually have a negative impact on their vision.

Most have also indicated that physical exercise seems to improve vision (subjectively). Stress can also include physical illness, trauma, loss of a loved one, loss of a job, financial stress, and relationship problems. These stress factors change the body chemistry as the Sympathetic Stress response is activated (sometimes acute and in some cases more chronic/habitual).

Changes in blood chemistry occur during periods of stress that cause neuroinflammation, oxidative stress, reduced peripheral blood flow, acidosis and weaken digestive function. Because stress responses can accelerate vision loss, stress management is an integral part of our program.

Some people are easier going and let things roll off their back. Then there are people who are more "Type-A" who just tend to run a bit more high strung and tend to be a little more emotionally charged. It is important to help ALL people manage stress and control their emotions so as to help preserve their vision.

Micro Acupuncture for Vision Preservation

Micro Acupuncture is one of the major acupuncture systems that I use for helping our patients improve and maintain healthy vision. This is a relatively new acupuncture system in which all the acupoints are located in the soles of feet and on palms of the hands. Acupuncture needles DO NOT get inserted into the eyes – which happens to be the most frequently asked question I get about the eye treatment.

Micro Acupuncture was originally developed in Denmark in the 1980's and then advanced by myself over the last 20 years.

The story about the guys who developed this method is that they were actually trying to treat arthritis. Some patients reported improved vision after the treatments and they soon found that it seemed to be very beneficial for eye conditions like glaucoma.

In 2016, I wrote and published the first book ever published on "Micro Acupuncture 48," which is available for acupuncturists who are interested in learning this acupuncture system.

We also use other acupuncture methods like traditional acupuncture, electroacupuncture, and low-level laser acupuncture.

Laser acupuncture is great for kids and for people who do not like needles. The cold laser has NO sensation and is good for those who have aversions to needles. The laser is used on the acupuncture points in place of needles, and it is just as effective. I have found laser acupuncture to be particularly beneficial for uncontrollable retinal bleeding and edema. We have also had a few documented cases in which acu-laser therapy lowered eye pressure.

How Acupuncture Benefits Vision

How does acupuncture help a patient diagnosed with Glaucoma?

First, acupuncture increases blood flow to the eyes and optic nerve. How do we know this? Ocular doppler and Ultra Sounds measure blood flow to the eye. The research studies I participated in and the acupuncture protocols that I developed for this research study (through Johns Hopkins University and NOVA Southeastern University) have demonstrated that acupuncture increases ocular blood flow.

I have identified specific acupuncture points that actually increase the blood flow to the eyes. This research has laid to rest the debate over whether or not acupuncture increases blood flow to the eyes. We now know that acupuncture can more definitely increase ocular circulation, bringing oxygen and nutrients to the eyes and optic nerve, as well as circulating out metabolic waste and carbon dioxide. Studies also show that acupuncture stimulates and lights up the visual cortex in the brain – the part of the brain that we use to process vision.

Acupuncture also stimulates the retina and optic nerve cells. It wakes up sleeping dormant nerve cells and helps facilitate cell repair of sick and/or damaged nerve cells.

Nerve cells need oxygen, glucose, and stimulation to remain functional. Some nerve cells are dead and others are just sleeping, dormant or inactive. Dead is dead, but we can charge up the dormant cells, heal sick/damaged cells and help preserve the healthy retinal and optic nerve cells.

Our Autonomic Nervous system has two branches – Sympathetic (fight or flight) and Parasympathetic (Relaxation and Recovery). Our acupuncture methods have a strong effect on regulating the autonomic nervous system by stimulating the parasympathetic, healing response.

Again, the Sympathetic response is your stress response and as we discussed, that can cause accelerated damage to your vision. The way our physiology and nervous system is wired, we simply can't heal and be stressed at the same time.

We're ONLY healing when we're in a Parasympathetic state - sleeping, relaxing, and meditating. We heal when we are engaged in hobbies and relaxing activities like gardening, drawing, dancing, etc. Activating the Parasympathetic system is a critical part of vision recovery and long-term vision preservation.

Objectives:

To Improve & Preserve Vision

In order to recover and preserve vision, the objective is to improve circulation and stimulate the optic nerve cells. Secondly, we may need to decrease inflammation, reduce oxidative stress, and manage any other underlying and/or contributing factors.

There's no one-size-fits-all treatment.

Yes, we want to control oxidative stress. Yes, we want to control inflammation. We want to help promote and maintain proper circulation to the optic nerve and to the retina. But there are other things going on with each individual person that we need to look at.

Maybe some have diabetes that is complicating the situation. Some might have a history of Lyme Disease which can adversely affect the optic and increase the rate of possible vision loss. Some have overwhelming emotional stress factors and others are on a lot of medication. Some have auto-immune conditions that are playing a role in their disease process. Everybody is going to be treated differently.

Again, the goal is to try to recover some lost vision to and then long-term vision preservation and neuroprotection.

The way we achieve that may differ with each patient.

I have been working hard to help move Ophthalmic Acupuncture into the realm of evidence-based medicine. Our research team worked hard to better understand the possible mechanisms of action and how acupuncture really works on ophthalmic diseases.

Mechanism of Vision Restoring
Using Acupuncture

There are four stages of cell health which involve the entire visual system - optic nerve, retina, and brain. Our eyes receive light and the light hits the retina; the light impulses are converted into electrical impulses and sends them to the brain for interpretation via the optic nerve.

There are four levels of cell health:

1-Normal

2-Dormant

3-Damaged

4-Dead

Normal cells are structurally sound, healthy and functioning. These photoreceptor cells receive light and send it to the brain in the form of electrical impulses.

Dormant means they're sleeping and inactive, like when your cell phone battery is dead. All you've got to do is charge it up, structurally it is fine. It just won't function on a dead battery, so we need to just charge it in order to work again.

Damaged cells are structurally abnormal and/or sick. The damage can be due to oxidative stress, poor oxygen, poor nutrition, inflammation, trauma, toxins, etc. These cells are sick and unhealthy, structurally impaired and poor function, but alive. They're not dead and they can be nursed back to health - it just takes time. How long? Current research suggests 8 to 15 months to rehab a sick or damaged nerve cell.

Nerves do not heal as fast as skin, hair, and nails, it takes more time. Science used to think that damaged nerves could not be repaired, but we know that is not true. It is just a slow regeneration that takes time.

How does this pertain to acupuncture treatment for glaucoma?

Generally, during the first few weeks of treatment, we are using acupuncture and supplements to activate dormant retinal and optic nerve cells. When the dormant cells become active, we may see some measurable improvement in the vision.

Over the next 8-15 months, we will be nursing sick cells back to health, regenerating them. After a year or so of treatment, we can pretty much assume that what we've recovered at that point is pretty much what we're able to recover. After that, it's all about long-term vision preservation.

Dead nerve cells, scar tissue, and fibrosis. Dead is dead and this is our fourth stage. We can't reincarnate dead tissue and bring it back to life.

The only person in history known to achieve such a feat as reanimation of dead tissue is the ever-popular Dr. Frankenstein. But seriously, once the tissue is dead, it's unfortunately gone forever.

When we do our initial vision testing on patients, the dormant cells, damaged cells, and dead cells are not functioning. There is simply no way to tell which are dead and which are dormant. The only way to tell dead from dormant is to provide a stimulus and see which cells respond and jump back into function.

Patients often ask, "How much vision can I get back?" I honestly don't have an answer to that because I have no way of knowing what the ratio of dead-to-dormant nerve cells is.

We simply don't how anyone will respond until we try to stimulate the cells and see how people respond.

The degree of improvement is in direct proportion to the ratio of dead to dormant nerve cells. The more dead cells, the less improvement there will be. The more dormant cells, the greater the chance for recovering lost vision. Simple concept, right?

20

Now let's take another example and look at two inactive bodies. One is sleeping; the other is in a coma. How do we know which it is which simply by looking? We don't!

How do we find out? By providing stimulus such as a bucket of water, air horn, shake them, kick them. We have to provide a stimulus and see which one wakes up. One is going to wake up; one is not after we've provided the right stimulus – which in this case is acupuncture.

Acupuncture wakes up dormant, sleeping retinal cells, optic nerve cells and the visual cortex of the brain.

Acupuncture provides the stimulus to stimulate the cells that are dormant, it rehabs the damaged cells and helps keep the normal cells healthy.

Again, our goal is the short-term recovery of lost vision and the long-term goal is to help you keep what you've got.

Stress Management for Vision Preservation

Stress management is very important for long-term vision preservation. Some people have a good predisposition to manage stress and seem to deal better with the adversity that life throws at them. Things just tend to roll off their backs and these folks tend to be relatively easy-going. Others may have been fortunate enough to have parents and family members who taught them how to manage stress from an early age. Some may have invested as adults in stress management training, self-help courses, meditation, or read some books (or audio books) to help us cope better with adversity and upset.

Generally, as we age and mature, we tend to care less about what other people think about us. We learn that we can't change others, we can only control ourselves and focus on controlling our own habits and emotions.

High levels of stress (acute or chronic) changes our internal biochemistry and systemic neurological functioning. These biochemical shifts if intense or frequent can often accelerate degenerative eye conditions like glaucoma.

Cortisol, adrenaline, and catecholamines are stress substances that flood the body when we are presented with a stressful situation. If we are in a chronically high-stressed state, this can be detrimental to our vision and accelerate neurodegeneration of the optic nerve associated with glaucoma.

Our Stress and Healing Response is regulated by our Autonomic Nervous system – Sympathetic and Parasympathetic Nervous System. Our bodies are wired to either be in a Sympathetic Stress state or Fight-Flight or in a Parasympathetic Rest-Repair-Recovery state. The way-out bodies are wired, we simply can't be stressed and heal at the same time.

If we are not sleeping, we are not recovering and regenerating. Taking sleep aids habitually, like Ambien every night (or alcohol), doesn't help the situation. We're passing out instead of sleeping. This is not the restful, restorative sleep we need for health and wellness and health preservation.

Here is a model that may help us to understand the stress response and what is happening. I learned this model from my good friend and colleague Dr. Marc Grossman, OD, LAc.

We have us or "me," and then we have our glaucoma/disease/stress or "it," - stress factor. Most of the time we are simply dealing and managing our "things" as they arise in our lives. "Me" is usually larger than "it," which is a relatively healthy and balanced state of existence.

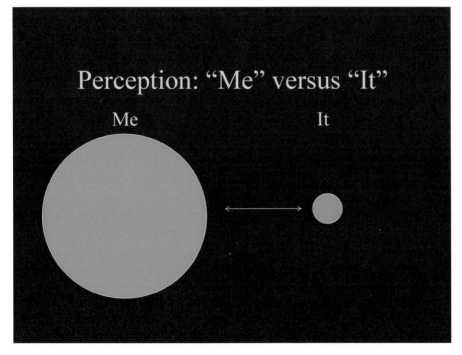

Sometimes these get switched. "Me" shrinks, and "It" seems larger than life, even overwhelming. "It" is vision loss, in this case, AMD or glaucoma or other eye issues. "It" is overwhelming. "It" is big and scary.

We can't deal with it so we react in a Fight or Flight Stress Response. Your eye doctor tells you, "Sorry, you have glaucoma and will lose your vision over time. We can try to slow the progression with eye drops and surgery to control your eye pressure but there are no guarantees."

High-stress responses and panic thoughts come into our minds like:

"How am I supposed to live?"

"How am I supposed to work?"

"How am I supposed to function?"

"Who will take care of me?"

Our goal is to identify that specific stress factor, neutralize the stress response and get ourselves back to an empowered and emotionally balanced state.

How do we get there? Through inquiry, education, and understanding of what we CAN and CANNOT control regarding the situation. We can be proactive and utilize integrative theories like medical eye drops, surgeries, acupuncture, eye exercises, nutrition and targeted supplements for glaucoma.

Most people will go to their eye doctor and are then told they have some type of eye condition like Glaucoma. Then they are told about the drugs and medical procedures that are recommended. Others are told that there is not much can be done for their condition, meaning that there is no conventional treatment at this point in time. Panic sets in! We tend to either run and hide in self-denial or we begin a process of self-educating to find out what is available outside conventional, mainstream medicine that may offer some benefits.

Through education and increasing what is available to us, we learn and increase our overall sense of relative power and control over the long-term preservation of one's vision. That will create a positive mindset and take us out of a state of "victim," and put us into Power.

How can we better manage stress? Once we educate ourselves on what options we have regarding our eye disease, we can look at other ways to help manage other stress-factors in our lives.

Meditation can be helpful to help us relax. There are also things like daily exercise and developing hobbies and interests. We also need to get the proper rest, sleep, and relaxation.

Mindfulness. What is on our minds most of the time? How do we talk to ourselves in our own heads and what do we focus on most of the time? Do we mull over the "doom and gloom" and how horrible life is and how much we are suffering?

Sometimes we have to learn to change our inner monolog and learn to say to ourselves, "I'm doing the best that I can." Or something like, "It's going to work out and be okay." Or even, "I can figure it out when I need to." Sometimes we think ourselves into a highly stressful emotional state of worry, anger, fear, anxiety, depression, etc. Although fleeting, emotions are normal, chronic, toxic emotions can tax our vision and overall health.

One of my favorite passages that I like to read when I feel stressed and consumed by negativity is the following:

(two wolves passage)

TWO WOLVES VIRTUES FOR LIFE

An old Cherokee is teaching his grandson about life.

"A fight is going on inside me," he said to the boy.
"It is a terrible fight and it is between two wolves. One is evil – he is anger, envy, sorrow, regret, greed, arrogance, self-pity, guilt, resentment, inferiority, lies, false pride, superiority, and ego."

He continued, "The other is good – he is joy, peace, love, hope, serenity, humility, kindness, benevolence, empathy, generosity, truth, compassion, and faith.

The same fight is going on inside you – and inside every other person, too."

The grandson thought about it for a minute and then asked his grandfather, "Which wolf will win?"

The old Cherokee simply replied, "The one you feed."

Other things that may help are reducing stimulants. Stimulants can get you jazzed up and feeling anxious. A lot of people consume a lot of coffee, soda, sugar, and alcohol which cause adrenaline surges and blood sugar fluctuations.

Stimulants don't give us true energy, they give us spurts of adrenaline, followed by a crash. In fact, they may even speed up neuro-degeneration and both dehydrate the body and cause excessive oxidative stress (accelerated aging).

Also, consider reducing sugar, alcohol, unnecessary medications, and smoking because they increase inflammation, acidosis, and oxidative stress.

Our Program

Most patients come in for one or two weeks of treatment for their initial series of treatment. We do vision testing before we begin and then we treat for a week and retest vision as a checkpoint.

The reason for the improvement in vision is because dormant cells become activated because of increased blood flow to the eye and neuro-stimulation.

Approximately 80-85 percent of patients respond positively and recover some lost vision during the first year of treatment. The more dormant cells, the more vision they recover. The more damage there is and the more advanced the case is less likely for improvement, but we can still help preserve vision. The earlier the stage, the easier it is to treat. The earlier we get our patients, the better the chances for long-term vision preservation.

Our patients receive an initial course of 10-20 acupuncture sessions and take a few recommended supplements to get the right nutrients to the eyes.

We also talk about nutrition and diet, home care instructions, lifestyle, maintenance, and follow-up. After we determine that there is a positive response, we can work on a long-term treatment plan for recovery and vision stabilization.

Regeneration of sick retinal cells can take 8 to 15 months. In that time, healthy new cells replace the sick or damaged ones. Our goal is to initially try to recover as much lost vision as possible. Long-term, the goal is preservation - to help you keep what you've got!

In terms of home care, we have patients who use supplements, use micro-current stimulation, improve diet, do eye exercises, and learn to better manage their stress.

If you have questions, please feel free to email me. The website is: www.acuvisionacupuncture.com

More About Dr. Rosenfarb and

His Integrative Approach

The brand name for our integrative approach is called *"AcuVision"* (www.acuvisonacupuncture.com) Acupuncture + Vision. This system is based on over two decades of clinical research and observation.

The AcuVision program incorporates different styles of acupuncture, herbs, supplements, eye exercises, nutrition, and lifestyle management.

Acupuncture is approximately 4,000 years old and there are different styles of acupuncture that have evolved over the millennia. I like to use the analogy of a tree. We refer to the trunk as the body of "acupuncture". The different branches of the tree represent the many styles of acupuncture that have developed over the last few thousand years.

All acupuncture systems have strong points, and they are all effective in some respects. For my purposes, I wanted to find out which systems were most effective for treating eye conditions. It has been many years of trial and error and we have by no means exhausted all acupuncture systems. I have figured out which systems seem to work best for certain eye conditions and which do not.

After years of trial and error, I kept and use the acupuncture methods that seem to show clear and relatively consistent results with my patients. I am constantly evolving and looking to improve our results which will be an ongoing process.

We have established highly effective acupuncture methods that demonstrate clinical efficacy. These acupuncture treatment strategies have also demonstrated efficacy in research trials with Johns Hopkins University and NOVA Southeast.

I began my education in this field in 1994 and studied Chinese Medicine at *Pacific College of Oriental Machine* in San Diego, California. After completing a four-year program, I received my Master in Traditional Oriental Medicine (MTOM) and went to China to continue my postgraduate studies. I also went on to study acupuncture in Europe, trying to find out as much as I could about different holistic-integrative methods for treating eye conditions.

After learning various acupuncture methods and systems, I experimented with a lot of them in my clinic to determine which offered the best results for degenerative eye conditions like Glaucoma and Optic Nerve Atrophy. Some of these methods I found to be very effective and others did not produce results. Over time, I retained those acupuncture methods that seemed to produce the best results and discarded those acupuncture systems that did not seem beneficial for my ophthalmic patients.

Over the years, my clinic has been somewhat of a laboratory of trying different Complementary-Alternative Medicine (CAM) treatment strategies including acupuncture, herbal medicine, vitamins and supplements,micro-current stimulation, color therapy, massage/eye exercises, essential oils, meditation, low-level laser therapy (LLLT), magnet therapy and ozone therapy. We've experimented with many forms of CAM therapies to figure out what gets the most consistent results. If the methods work, then we keep them and if not, we drop them.

One of the great things about treating vision is that we can easily measure efficacy and response with standard, ophthalmic vision testing. We simply take a baseline vision test before commencing acupuncture treatment (acuity, visual field, contrast, eye pressure, etc.) and then retest after a series of treatments to confirm improvement. There is either a positive, objective measurable improvement or there is not. There can be noted subjective benefits - improvements that the patients report from treatment. After we confirm that a patient is a "responder", we will continue to monitor improvements until the patient plateaus and the vision stabilizes.

I've written and published several books, articles and research reports on Acupuncture & Chinese Medical Ophthalmologic conditions. These are available for both patients and healthcare professionals. Over many years of doing field research, I have accumulated and compiled information and the treatment of degenerative eye conditions. I organized the data wrote my first book in 2003 called, Healing Your Eyes with Chinese Medicine.

GLAUCOMA MANAGEMENT

Most cases of glaucoma that I work with have elevated intraocular pressure (IOP). I see other forms as well, including normal tension glaucoma (NTG), pseudoexfoliation glaucoma and steroid-induced glaucoma. Most patients are on IOP meds and/or have had procedures to try to help control the IOP.

The focus of Conventional Ophthalmic Glaucoma Specialists is to control the IOP and keep it low to reduce the stress placed on the optic nerve. Elevated eye pressure can lead to optic nerve damage/atrophy progressive vision loss. Glaucoma specialists work to control eye pressure - and treatment is isolated and restricted to controlling eye pressure. There is a host of surgical procedures and medications to lower and control eye pressure.

In many cases, controlling IOP is simply not enough to preserve vision. The health and function of the optic nerve declines and patients continue to lose vision. This is a major problem!

Conventional Ophthalmology has gotten very good (in most cases) in terms of helping to reduce IOP. This specific risk factor must be controlled to help preserve the optic nerve. Unfortunately, for many, controlling IOP is not enough to prevent progressive vision loss and optic nerve degeneration.

How do we know that controlling IOP is not always enough to prevent vision loss?

We know this because many glaucoma patients are on IOP lowering eye drops and have had surgical procedures (SLT, trabeculectomy, iridotomy) and the eye pressure is relatively low and controlled.

Glaucoma patients continue to lose vision over time even with controlled eye pressure.

MAKING GOOD DECISIONS

At this point, you can make a few decisions about your vision:

1. You can consider the information in this book and continue to do what you are doing and hope you don't lose more vision.

2. You can do some more research about what we do, perhaps watch some of our free videos on our YouTube Channel.

3. You can call or email us for more information.

4. You're interested and open to trying treatment to see if it works.

5. You fully resonate with our message and want to go all-in and decide to be proactive with your vision.

If you are looking for more information feel free to give us a call

(908) 928-0060

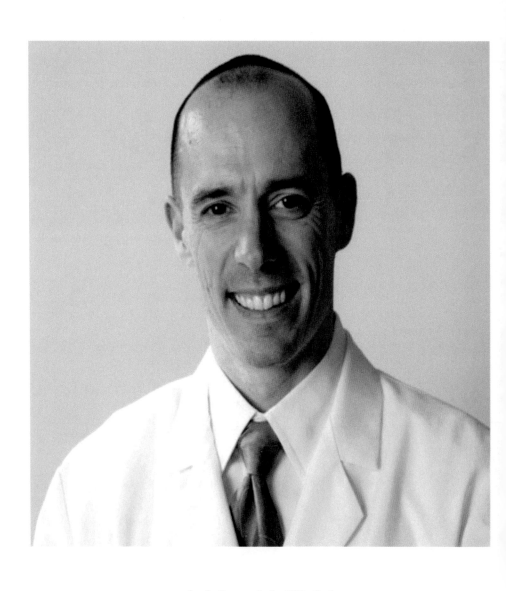

Andy Rosenfarb, ND, L.Ac.

332 South Ave East

Westfield, NJ 07090

908-928-0060

www.acuvisionacupuncture.com

Made in the USA
Las Vegas, NV
08 August 2024

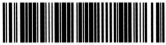

93538482R00029